The Scars of War

Paul Tribus

 Unless otherwise identified, Scripture quotations are from The King James Version of the Bible.

Companion Press
P.O. Box 310
Shippensburg, PA 17257-0310

ISBN 1-56043-493-7

For Worldwide Distribution
Printed in the U.S.A.

Dedication

This book is dedicated to all the veterans of every war, and to the families, who become part of the war without ever enlisting.

Acknowledgements

I would like to acknowledge all the ministers who have poured into my life over the last 20 years, my wife Joanne, and two children Michele, and Michael who helped me to recall a lot of the material in this book, and who patiently endured as I put this very painful part of my life into print. Also I want to acknowledge Cynthia Ellenwood who helped with the research and spent many hours in prayer in seeking the Lord for His purpose and timing for this book.

Table of Contents

Foreword

Desert Storm has been billed as a classical American success story. Our nation has been enjoying an "all time high" in national pride and world esteem. We have celebrated, marched and waved flags and yellow ribbons from coast to coast, and rightly so—our fighting men and women deserve our respect and appreciation.

But there is another side of war, the personal trauma that accompanies death on a wholesale scale. At its worst, it tears the soul and spirit of man and leaves him irreparably damaged like the tortured souls who returned from Vietnam.

Even at its best, like the pristine textbook war in the Gulf, there is an irreversible change in the human spirit that can't be glossed over by patriotic speeches or erased by the support of friends and family.

The scars are deep and time doesn't heal them completely. Every new war reopens the wounds...and there is always another war. The Bible says that there will be "wars and rumors of wars" until the end of this age. We must find ways to deal with the pain and cope with the effects of war.

I know of no better time for a book such as this one, and no better person to address these issues than Reverend Paul Tribus. The things he shares come from personal experience as a veteran of Vietnam, as a pastor and as a counselor to vets and their families.

I have known Paul for nearly two decades. I have witnessed the life-changing effects of the principles he shares in this book. I have seen lives saved and families rescued from the brink of destruction.

This book is a book of hope and healing. It is also a book of truth and answers which satisfy. It will minister to vets, but beyond that it will give families and friends, pastors and counselors the means to help the ones they love.

It is my hope and prayer that many will find the peace they seek in these pages and in the process become acquainted with the Prince of peace.

Bishop John Gimenez
Pastor of Rock Church
Bishop of Rock Ministerial Fellowship
National Chairman of Washington
for Jesus, 1980 and 1988

Introduction

There are places in Vietnam where the elephant grass is so dense you scarcely can see in front of you. Even the sunlight has trouble getting through it. For the last twenty years, the American public has been struggling through its own jungle—a choking undergrowth of lies about Vietnam. Thanks to the persistence of the media, the people received almost no true light on the reasons we vets fought and died there. Instead, they were overwhelmed with horror stories about evil soldiers and conniving generals.

The Vietnam vet, twenty years later, now faces a different kind of war. No longer is he struggling through rice paddies, being pinned down under mortar fire or sleeping in a foxhole and hoping he will awaken one more time. Today the vet fights a battle raging in his mind.

Vietnam put confusion in the vet's mind and spirit. With one set of rules his country asked him to go to war. Now he is asked to live by another set of rules. Whenever he requests help there is so much red tape that he feels everyone is fighting against him. Even when he feels a glimmer of hope he is disappointed, because he gets no lasting solutions. Parades and memorials help for a little while. Handouts and attention to outward problems bring some relief. What the vet needs, however, is deep ministry to his heart and mind. He needs effective weapons to fight this new war—spiritual weapons that work.

This battle is real. The veterans know it. They also know that it involves the people close to them. They no longer fight alone in a distant country. They have brought this war to their wives, children, family, friends, employers, priests and ministers.

America cannot turn its back on this problem and hope it will go away. We need to resolve it by refusing to walk on the tangled pathway others made for us.

This book deals with the war in several different ways.

First, because I am a veteran, I understand the scars of war that no one sees. Even after I became a Christian and a pastor, I still went through some difficult times. Christians are not exempt.

I also look at the war from the viewpoint of history. Why were we there? What are the real answers? We have gotten the run-around long enough. Now is the hour when we must square our shoulders and "Stand Tall".

I try to give families and friends of vets some answers. They need to know how to stand tall as well.

This book is for all veterans and for all who have become a part of this war, the war of the mind.

We must deal boldly with the issues because it takes backbone to stand tall. We need the strength that comes from understanding what happens in our lives today and happened twenty years ago.

The last few chapters of this book take a closer look at the war in the Persian Gulf. It is like an older brother helping his younger sibling. Because I have been in war, I believe I have some keen insight to help the men and women from the war in the Gulf. War is a terrible thing physically, emotionally and spiritually. It does not matter if it is in a rice paddy or a desert; extreme pressure is put upon the mind and emotions.

I can provide answers in this book only because the Lord has enlightened me and because of the experiences I have been allowed to have. They were very painful, but if I can help someone, it all will be worth it.

But this book is more than a testimony of one vet's experience. It addresses the problems any war brings and the problems that remain long after the war ceases. It brings godly answers. I hope it will bring light, revelation and hope to you.

Chapter 1

The War Rages On

The phone was ringing. As a church pastor in Pennsylvania, I was trying to make final preparations for the evening service. I didn't want to sound annoyed, but I had a lot on my mind. "Hello," I said testily.

"Hey, Tribus! It's your buddy, Sonny!" exploded a familiar Texas drawl in my ear. It had been about seven years since Sonny and I fought together in 'Nam, but once in awhile we got together by phone.

"Hey! How're you doin', Sonny?" I asked. He was a great guy, but I hoped this call wouldn't be one of our long conversations.

"Believe it or not," he said, "I'm not too far away from you. We were just free-ridin' through D.C. and I thought I'd drop by if you weren't too busy."

"That would be great," I said, cringing, "but this isn't the best time for me. I hope you understand. I've got church tonight and then I'm tied up tomorrow. Why don't we make it another time?"

"Hey, buddy, no problem," Sonny said. He made a few light remarks about how great it would be to see me, but he didn't say it was urgent or anything. He hung up soon afterwards and I went about my work, "the Lord's work," not realizing how badly I had blown it.

I never would have admitted it then, but I was beginning to struggle with all my personal relationships. Like many other Vietnam vets, a war still raged inside me.

In country (the term for Vietnam) I was not wounded physically. I was wounded on the inside. But I never asked for help because I thought I could handle everything by myself. Vietnam had taught us to survive on our own. We went everywhere alone: boot camp, training, combat and rest and relaxation. Sure, there were always other people around, but even when we shared a foxhole we tried not to care too much about the other guys.

In those long, boring days between enemy actions, I spent hours alone with my thoughts about the war. After I got home, I tried not to think about it at all. Instead, I pushed everything down inside.

I thought I had found the magic formula for solving my Vietnam problem back in my early twenties, when I became a

Christian, started a family and began to pastor a church. Yet all the time something terrible was happening inside me because of those thoughts I had pushed down and suppressed. I thought I could use religion like a Band-Aid. Band-Aids don't work on mortal wounds. I didn't know it at the time, but all the weapons for winning that inner war were available to me, and yet, I never picked them up and used them.

The last few years have been the hardest ones of my life, but they also have been the best. I finally have begun to understand that the war raging inside us is not hopeless. There are answers. That is why I wrote this book. I know how vets can win.

Starting a New Life

Twice in my life I have seen a man severely beaten, once when I was in the service and once after I became a pastor. In both cases the person's face was marred and swollen so badly that he was unable to see.

As a Christian, I know that Jesus was beaten, too. But as He lay in the tomb and the grubs came to eat off His flesh, something miraculous happened. He received a healing from the Father. After the resurrection He still had the scars in his hands, feet and side, but there is no record of any signs of the beatings. He was no longer disfigured.

You may feel as if your life has been ruined by beatings. You may be convinced that no one cares about you. Maybe you feel that you barely exist in a place of death and that there is no hope for you. If that is your situation, regardless of what you believe about Jesus right now, consider what it could mean for you to come back to life again as a whole person, without a trace of disfigurement. You may always have a few scars; after all, they confirm what you have gone through. But those scars have no power to hurt you. They can become scars of healing, to be shared with others.

Whatever your background or beliefs, if you want to turn your life around, the most important step you can take is to believe in the Jesus of the tomb.

The Needs of Vets

News about Southeast Asia almost vanished from the American media after South Vietnam was overrun with Communists in 1975. Vets, for the most part, decided to keep their opinions and experiences to themselves. Several years later a group of dedicated people got together and built a war memorial in Washington, D.C., dedicated on Veteran's Day in 1982. It became possible to reopen the subject of the war.

As a result, countless movies, books and conversations about the Vietnam War have sprung up from Congress to college campuses. In the process, more than a few observers have tried to determine what happened with the Vietnam vets that didn't happen in previous wars and why Vietnam vets have more needs. I have read what they say and some of their points are right, but other factors seem to have escaped their attention. However, for now let me tell you what I think vets need.

Vets need one another. Those who never spent any time in country do not understand what it was like. Vets who have made peace with their pasts, or are at least willing to try, have a great deal to offer one another.

What was it like? Almost from the first moment a soldier arrived he was hot, sweaty and in fear for his life. Most of them were under twenty years old and hardly knew what life was all about. By the time they went home, twelve or thirteen months later (if they didn't get wounded sooner), they were totally changed. They had done things that would have been unthinkable a few months earlier: taken lives, gotten drunk, had fist fights, gone to prostitutes. A few even had committed atrocities against women and children.

A lot of vets never have forgiven themselves for what they did in Vietnam. Their guilt is buried deep within them. If they want to be whole again, **vets need to stop punishing themselves.**

Twenty years have passed, but some vets still are afraid that they could commit those acts again. It does not have to happen. Help is available twenty-four hours a day. **Vets need a Power greater than themselves.**

Sometimes vets even feel guilty for legitimate actions done in the line of duty. They have lost their understanding of what communism is and why it threatens America. Many never knew why they were there in the first place. So they join the chorus of bitterness.

For twenty years vets have accepted condemnation from people who have no understanding of the war. It is time for vets to stand tall again. They accomplished a lot. **Vets need to be proud of their acts of service.**

When in the bush, you were part of a team of three or four Marines who made up a squad. For a few months you ate together, slept together, fought the same enemy and battled the same environment. You had no TV, no movies and no entertainment, except for a rare USO show. After awhile, you got to know a lot about one another.

The guys I spent the most time with were Rudy, Ted and Sonny. Rudy was Hispanic, Ted was black and Sonny was white, like me. By the time Ted left for home, Rudy and Sonny were wounded and I can still remember Ted, with tears in his eyes, telling me to be careful.

Vets can harp on the few racist incidents that occurred under stress if they want to, but it will not bring them peace. It will not further the cause of racial justice. If they want wholeness, **vets need to recapture the good times.**

About all we had to look forward to each day were our meals. But one time we got stuck in such an intense combat zone that we had no supplies for a week, not even cans of C-rations.

Those who had extra food stockpiled, like cans of peanut butter or cake, were selling them for five or ten dollars a piece. Finally, even those reserves ran out. Still no helicopters could get in to us.

We had to keep moving because of the danger, but we were getting weaker. Marches were bad enough in the 110 to 120 degree heat, but without supplies they were almost unbearable. Tempers flared. Men pledged to tell their congressmen about this inhumane treatment. Others griped, "We're out here risking our necks. Why can't the backups do their jobs?" Vets still expect the government to solve all their problems. That is impossible. **Vets need to look beyond the government for their recovery.**

After awhile, we lost even our common sense. When out on patrol, we were fired on by a sniper. Instead of immediately diving for cover, we all turned and charged him. It was insane.

Today vets may not be physically hungry like we were then, but they have a gnawing hunger in their souls and spirits for inner peace. It eats away at them until they do irrational things like attacking their wives and children—not necessarily with physical violence but with emotional abuse that is just as damaging. I have struggled with that myself.

If vets want to become well, they need to realize that the anger and pain they feel is often unrelated to the events that trigger those feelings. They need to find out what actually is wrong with them and be healed. **Vets need healing of body, soul and spirit.**

After we charged the sniper, three more days passed with absolutely no food. Finally a helicopter managed to drop a pallet of Campbell's Soup for us. One can apiece. I can still remember how we sat and looked tenderly at our own personal dinner. We opened them carefully, leaving part of the lid attached for a handle. Then we set them up with the portable heat-tab we each carried along in our packs. Hot chicken noodle soup coming up.

Sonny set his can on a slight slope, then reached back for a spoon. That was his mistake. By the time he had reached back, the whole can had tipped over and the broth was making little channels in the dirt. I'll never forget the look on his face. He simply could not believe it.

Suddenly, Sonny reached down, scooped up those gritty noodles and stuffed them in his mouth, dirt and all. We burst out laughing. **Vets need to laugh about their problems.** And that is perhaps the hardest of all to do.

The Spiritual Needs of Vets

On my first day in Vietnam, several Marines who had been there for awhile helped show us newcomers the ropes. That night we got hit. There was a heart-stopping shout: "Incoming!" then the whistle of enemy mortars.

Suddenly the NVA (North Vietnamese Army) charged up the hill and opened fire. We returned fire and threw hand grenades, then we returned mortar fire. The whole thing happened so fast I didn't have time to think about it until it was over. That skirmish lasted only thirty minutes, but it stayed with me all night long. All I could think was, "This is my first day. I have 394 left. How will I ever make it? When will I get killed?" The thought of my death haunted me. **Vets need to learn how to deal with death.**

One night some months later we saw activity just ahead of us and went on a hundred percent alert. Spot, up front, had been with me for my first three months in 'Nam, including a stretch in the DMZ (demilitarized zone between North and South Vietnam). With us trailing cautiously behind him, he waded into one of the swamps that always blocked our path and took a look. It seemed to be a helmet just floating in the water, but when he picked it up he found something else—a live Viet Cong officer. We grabbed him.

Before anyone else arrived, we looked in his pack. It was one of the laws of the jungle that you took what you could get and no one was the wiser. This time we couldn't believe our good luck. The pack was filled with money, North Vietnamese money. The enemy we had captured was a paymaster coming down to pay the troops. We took the money and hid it for ourselves. When questioned later, we denied everything.

That night disaster hit. About supper time we were attacked and pinned down. The battle raged on for hours. When the smoke cleared, Spot was dead. In one horrible moment his body had been blown apart, and the money along with him.

Battlefield deaths are a terrible ordeal. First you lose a friend in a brutal and devastating event. Then you must leave the body out there until it is safe to retrieve it. When you reach what is left of your buddy you have to take care of his remains yourself. You grieve for the family and friends he told you about. You have an intense fear that you might be next but know you must keep fighting.

That night I stayed up all night alone and cried and cried.

It was agonizing to try to survive all the killing, the fights and the terrifying nights, but it also did something to souls and spirits when soldiers stole, lied and committed adultery. After awhile, you began to call evil good and good evil. Your whole thinking process became muddled.

There is only one way to clear up that kind of thinking—definite standards of right and wrong. Those who were captured and forced to live in prison camps had a strong code of ethics. Sometimes that code was all that kept them going. They knew what their limits were and how much the others needed to depend on them. **Vets need to take a strong moral stand.**

Some people will say that vets won't listen if I talk about moral standards and God, but I don't believe it. Maybe there were no longer prayer and Bible readings in high school, but we knew about God and we talked to Him in those foxholes.

I remember how we used to read the Bible together before it got dark. Psalm 91 was a favorite of ours. By the time I got home I could quote the whole psalm. You probably have heard verses like these:

> *He that dwelleth in the secret place of the most High shall abide under the shadow of the Almighty...Thou shalt not be afraid for the terror by night; nor for the arrow that flieth by day...A thousand shall fall at thy side, and ten thousand at thy right hand; but it shall not come nigh thee...Because thou hast made the LORD, which is my refuge, even the most High, thy habitation.*
>
> Psalm 91:1,5,7,9

Imagine four Marines, after digging a foxhole or getting ready for night patrol, self-consciously pulling a Bible out of the pack and carefully unwrapping it. (Everything had to be wrapped in plastic to keep it from getting wet.) Then we would take off our helmets and bow our heads to God as we read. We didn't understand all of it, but with great reverence we read and asked that God's protection be with us. **Vets need God's help and protection.**

Most of the experts in Post Traumatic Stress Disorder (PTSD) say, "We know Vietnam vets have a problem and we are trying to find a cure. Just give us more time." I say we have waited long enough. We need answers that work. Vets still suffer from Vietnam because of their physical and emotional injuries, but they also have allowed the Vietnam experience to wound their spirits. The answer is not "religion". That did not work for me and it will not work for you. I am talking about the same kind of deep healing for your spirit that you want for your body, mind and emotions.

Maybe this story will explain my meaning. Jesus once encountered ten lepers (Luke 17:12-19). For years this terrible disease affected their lives. Maybe you can identify with the way they lived: always staying away from people, feeling unclean, trying to hide from those who mocked and tormented them and feeling at ease only with other lepers, day after day, night after night, for weeks, months and years. They could not visit their families. They had to cover their faces and hands and cry out, "Unclean! Unclean!" to everyone who passed by them.

When the lepers cried to Jesus for mercy, He answered by sending them to the priest to confirm what He was about to do. As they went on their way, a miracle happened. Suddenly they were healed. Can you imagine it? As they walked, fingers grew back, scales fell off and new flesh appeared where once was only sores. They were healed physically.

Ten lepers were cleansed, but only one turned around and said thanks. Only one had a grateful heart. When Jesus saw that, He said to the leper, "Thy faith hath made thee whole." Ten men were healed physically, but only the one who thanked God was made completely whole.

If you go to a VA hospital, the medical personnel can probably heal your body and even may offer you some help for your mind. But if you want to be **whole**, you will have to do something else–have a grateful heart. **Vets need to thank God for all He has brought them through.**

Once something wounds your spirit, only God can fix it. When that leper turned back to say thanks, I am sure he still had scars and memories from his years as a leper. But because he had been made whole, he had a new life in spite of them.

Do you remember what it was like to slog through those rice paddies in Vietnam? No matter how much you wanted to move faster, you had to take one step at a time. Maybe you are tired of causing problems for yourself and for others and are looking for quick answers. Be patient. Walk through the rice paddies of your life with me for awhile. I want to show you what actually happened in Vietnam and why your action there was so important. Then I want to help you overcome your fears, fix broken relationships and find fresh enthusiasm for your life and work.

Many people have scars in their lives. These scars are from war, from divorce, from drugs and from alcohol. If you can get healed, you can help not only yourself but also those other people. You can tell them how you were made whole.

Chapter 2

How Did We Get in this Mess?

"How did I get in this mess?" As I struggled through the rice paddies or lay awake in the foxholes at night, I often asked myself that question.

It all started one night when I was fooling around at the local hangout, the Purple Haze, with a bunch of the guys. It had been almost a year since I graduated from high school in Swoyersville, Pennsylvania, but I still had no plans, no sense of direction for my life.

We were sitting there talking about nothing when my buddy Mike suddenly said to me, "Why don't you join the Marines? Hey, I dare you! I'm doing it."

Why the Marines? I don't know, but the next day I found myself at the recruiter's and he was signing me up. That was 1968! A war was on, even if it wasn't called a war. People were getting killed in Vietnam. It was some dare.

It was hard on my Mom, as she had counted on me to help pay the bills and work around the house. My Dad had died three years earlier.

When the bus drove us into boot camp at Parris Island it turned out we weren't reporting just for a new job. We were being thrown through the gate that separated boyhood from manhood. We never had a chance to say good-bye. Our minds were full of fear, but we would die rather than say so. A lot of things we learned to stuff inside us in the months to come. For some of us, that continual pushing down eventually would kill us just as surely as a VC land mine.

That night at Parris Island we learned pretty fast that if we wanted to stay out of trouble we better shut up, take orders and keep moving. Before the bus had stopped rolling, a drill instructor marched across the road and headed straight for us. He looked mean and he didn't waste time on anything like "Hi, fellas, how're ya doin'?" He started barking orders and we started jumping. We didn't stop until one o'clock in the morning.

Everybody fell into bed and drifted off. Crash! It was 4 a.m. and the drill instructor was throwing on the light switch and smashing empty trash cans across the floor. Bodies went flying, either jumping up like scared rabbits or being thrown out of bed.

Welcome to the United States Marine Corps.

Training was anything but glorious. We were treated like dogs and it never let up. One day about two weeks into our training the drill instructor came into the barracks and talked to us real nicely for a change. "You guys have tried us out for awhile," he said sweetly. "It's our policy to give you a chance at this point to give up and go home, if that's what you want. Anybody who wants to quit just come up to my desk."

Everybody looked around at each other. It was really quiet. Then we looked at the floor. It was time to decide and nobody wanted to admit what he was thinking. Finally, about five guys self-consciously walked up to the desk.

"Is there anybody else?" he asked. I was having one giant struggle inside me. I wanted so badly to go up there too, but I couldn't make up my mind. I hate pressure decisions. "Last chance," he called. One more "recruit" went up.

"Well," said the sergeant. "You guys want to go home?" Then his whole tone of voice changed. The wolf came snarling out of his sheep's clothing. "Are you mama's boys?" he said mockingly. "Can't you take it?" They turned beet red. "Did you really think we were going to let you go home?" I was dying with embarrassment for them. It could have been me up there.

"Get down and do fifty push-ups," he barked. "Then stand in front of these other recruits and let them see the little cowards who want to go home because they can't take it." I was so glad I didn't go up there. Boy, was I glad. At that moment I felt the most incredible relief that I had passed a test.

It was tough, but it was all part of the mental and physical training. Get tough. That was the point. Get tough. We were about to face life and death situations we couldn't even imagine. Somebody had to convince us to quit looking for a way to retreat and pay attention to fighting the battle. It was hell, but it did something for us that none of those exempted war resisters on their college campuses ever experienced.

The anti-war folks destroyed some of us with their contempt when we returned. Yet a lot of us twenty years later still can say, "Yeah, man. I went to Vietnam. I served my country. I didn't understand all of it, but you know what? I'd do it again."

A funny thing has happened since then, too. Some of those grown-up rebels realized they were wrong for hating us and calling us liars and baby killers. Some have publicly apologized to the vets. They know now that they didn't bring peace to America.

All in all it has given some of us the courage to go back, look at the war itself and try to find out what really happened in Vietnam. I want to tell you what I found out.

What Really Happened in Vietnam

When I arrived in country I found out real fast that it was not rumors I had been hearing about death and destruction. This place was dangerous. It was also hot.

As we got off the plane the heat almost knocked us over, it was so intense. We were taken by helicopter out into the bush. What a view! Most of the thick jungle undergrowth was still there in those days. Agent Orange was yet a few years away.

As we unloaded Captain Smith approached us. "You'll be assigned to Echo Company," he told us.

Somebody said, "Sir, our orders read Fox Company."

"That was before the Third Platoon of Echo Company was wiped out," he said matter-of-factly. "Everyone was killed or wounded. You're the new Third Platoon."

My first day in Vietnam.

Most Americans have almost no understanding of the Vietnam War. They have taken sides—and violently defended their positions—based on misconceptions and inaccurate information. Most people have relied on television and newspaper reporters for the whole truth. These, at best, only can offer partial truths. Their work is to report daily happenings. They don't have time to verify everything. They also have very definite opinions that filter through their news. According to every poll, the media reveal themselves as overwhelmingly against the war. In fact, they disagree with most of the American public on a great number of issues, yet they have been allowed to shape everyone's thinking. Here are a few facts people probably didn't read in the newspaper, see on TV or find in the movies full of foul language.

Facts about Vietnam

Vietnam is a country located in the Far East area called Indochina. Originally the offspring of India and China, Indochina was conquered by France in the nineteenth century and added to its empire. Indochina included the states of Vietnam, Laos and Cambodia.

As with any colonized people, the citizens of Vietnam began to resent the French and to plot ways of gaining their independence. Of the numerous nationalist organizations, the most powerful was led by Ho Chi Minh. Ho was an unrelenting member of the Communist Party and the Comintern, the internationalist arm of the Party allied with Moscow. Although he once offered to renounce his affiliation with the Communist Party in return for American assistance in overthrowing the French, his future actions revealed the emptiness of his promises.

Ho's admirers, including some Americans who thought all liberation wars were the same, considered him a Vietnamese George Washington. That only proved they knew neither Washington nor Ho. Washington was a man of the highest moral standards, who sought guidance from God and from his fellow man in all his decisions. Ho Chi Minh was a ruthless atheist whose only goal was power. He wanted to rule Vietnam as a communist state regardless of the people's wishes or the cost in ruined lives.

In 1940 a new factor complicated the situation. The Japanese occupied northern Indochina while France itself was occupied by the Germans. In March 1945, the Japanese dissolved the French government throughout Indochina and declared Vietnam independent. Emperor Bao Dai pledged cooperation with Japan.

After the atomic bombs were dropped on Hiroshima and Nagasaki and Japan surrendered, Vietnam was once again in turmoil. Emperor Bao Dai abdicated. The Americans, French, British and Chinese all were involved in various parts of that tiny country. Murders and insurrections occurred constantly. The Viet Minh (at first composed of both communists and other nationalists but later dominated by the Communist Party) began guerilla warfare. The French alternately agreed to independence and refused to grant it. In hopes of rallying the Vietnamese people away from Ho, a new government was established, headed by former emperor Bao Dai.

By 1950 there were two distinct Vietnams. The North was run by Ho and the Communist Party and recognized by China and the Soviet Union. The South was headed by Bao Dai, with the Western nations jockeying for influence.

After a series of complicated events, on May 8, 1954, the Viet Minh defeated the French at Dien Bien Phu. Bao Dai appointed Ngo Dinh Diem as premier of South Vietnam while he himself remained head of state. On July 21, the Geneva Accords were signed. It included a provision to divide Vietnam along the 17th parallel until reunification elections could be held.

In 1955 the United States began direct aid to the Vietnamese. In the past aid had been given via the French. At first this aid was rather limited. But by 1953, under President Eisenhower, American funds were supplying eighty percent of the French effort to subdue Vietnam. Although Eisenhower had said originally that Indochina was not strategically important, it later became apparent to him that it would create a "domino effect" if it fell. Other nations in the region then would fall to communism as well.

In 1955 a national referendum was held in South Vietnam. As a result, the somewhat unstable Bao Dai was deposed and Diem became president. On December 12, the U.S. Consulate in Hanoi was closed. The national elections specified in the Geneva Accords never were held. Instead, until 1975, "voting" was done by machine guns and land mines.

Each U.S. president had the lofty goal of helping the helpless and of protecting the world from communism. Each one made serious errors in the methods of achieving that goal.

Truman sent the first Americans to Vietnam but his concerns about Europe clouded the issue. He never repudiated French colonialism or endorsed Vietnam's independence. This departure from principle later set the stage for the Soviet and Chinese Communists, through their leader Ho Chi Minh, to appear as deliverers to the Vietnamese people.

Eisenhower aided the French and later the Vietnamese people directly. He tried to pick up the complicated pieces left after the Geneva Accords, but his attention was diverted to the war in Korea.

Kennedy pledged in his inaugural address, "Let every nation know that we shall pay any price, bear any burden, meet any hardship, support any friend, oppose any foe to assure the survival and the success of liberty." Little did he know how impossible it would be to keep that pledge, or the compromises that he would make.

Johnson was haunted by his desire to declare war on poverty and by his wish to conclude successfully the war in Vietnam. His personal involvement in complex military decisions and his reluctance to commit sufficient funds caused the war effort to stagnate.

Nixon had been involved in Vietnam since his vice-presidency under Eisenhower. Through his efforts China and the Soviet Union participated in the extrication of American forces, but his unconscionable practices related to Watergate destroyed his ability to complete what the U.S. had started in Vietnam.

Through every presidential succession the Communists kept up a continual barrage of lies to the Vietnamese, about the evil American "imperialists" who wanted to destroy them and steal their land. Thus it is not surprising that so many were willing to fight us. What is remarkable is the number of Vietnamese who refused to believe the propaganda and looked to the Americans as their only hope for freedom.

The South Vietnamese wanted us to free them from their communist oppressors. But we only gave them implements of war, never what they needed: the implements of peace. Because of a series of disastrous decisions by both Vietnamese and American policy makers, the South Vietnamese people never formed a strong enough bond with one another to fight onward for the total victory. Even when the Americans won the war for them, they were unable to maintain the peace. They didn't understand the basic principles of one nation under God. They didn't need a clone of our government; they needed to understand why we remain free and prosperous while other nations rise and fall.

Although Ho Chi Minh died before the final communist takeover of South Vietnam, his totalitarian leadership was so strong that it forged a North Vietnamese people bound together like iron. Without scruples concerning human rights, they forced all who disagreed to join their movement. Without a godly nation to the south to repel them, they proved invincible.

Myths about the Vietnam War

Ever since we went to Vietnam, a number of myths about our involvement continually have resurfaced. These damaged the war effort, but even more importantly, they disrupted our national unity. Even today, both vets and non-vets quote these myths to justify their hold on their bitterness. It is time to stop using these myths as clubs to hurt one another, for in the process we hurt ourselves.

Because Richard M. Nixon resigned in disgrace, his insights into the Vietnam conflict often are discredited. However, in his book **No More Vietnams** he compiled an important list that many Americans need to re-examine. He may not be correct on every point, but most of them have solid documentation.

Here are the common myths that Nixon listed in his book (pp. 9-10):

- The Vietnam War was a civil war.
- Ho Chi Minh was a nationalist first and a Communist second and had the support of a majority of the people of Vietnam, North and South.
- Ngo Dinh Diem was a puppet of the French colonialist.
- The National Liberation Front was a revolutionary movement independent of North Vietnam.
- The Viet Cong won the hearts and minds of villagers through humanitarian policies.

- The Geneva Declaration of 1954 legally bound Diem's government and the United States to unify the two halves of Vietnam through elections.
- The agreements in 1962 "neutralizing" Laos prevented the widening of the war.
- The Buddhist protests in 1962 against Diem resulted from religious repression.
- The Johnson administration was the first to send American troops into combat in Vietnam.
- Most American soldiers were addicted to drugs, guilt-ridden about their role in the war, and deliberately used cruel and inhumane tactics.
- American blacks constituted a disproportionate number of the combat casualties.
- The United States lost the war militarily.
- The Communist Tet Offensive of 1968 was a military defeat for the United States.
- U.S. secret bombing in 1969 and ground attacks on the Communist bases in Cambodia in 1970 were responsible for bringing the Communists into power in Cambodia in 1975.
- It was a calculated policy of the United States to bomb civilian targets in North Vietnam.

- The percentage of civilian deaths in the Vietnam War was higher than in other wars.
- American POWs were treated humanely by the North Vietnamese.
- The anti-war demonstrations in the United States shortened the war.
- The Paris peace agreements of 1973 were a cynical attempt to provide the United States with a "decent interval" between the withdrawal of its forces and the collapse of South Vietnam.
- The United States could have struck the same deal in 1969 as it did in 1973.
- The domino theory has been proved false.
- Life is better in Indochina now that the United States is gone.

The belief in these lies about Vietnam continues to divide our country and keeps vets from the recognition they deserve.

From 1954 to 1973, American aid and military forces were responsible for protecting at least a segment of the Vietnamese population from the attack dogs of the Communist Party. As Jesus said, "Greater love hath no man than this, that a man lay down his life for his friends" (John 15:13). American GIs didn't even know the Vietnamese before they went over there, but they laid down their lives for them.

When Vietnam was overrun in 1975, no longer was there anyone to speak up for the unalienable human rights granted by the Creator. No one was left in Vietnam to argue for freedom of religion or of the press. Americans in Vietnam saved many lives. Communists in Vietnam destroyed them.

That is why we fought.

We did not lose the war militarily; we lost politically. With the war in the Persian Gulf, we knew the cause and objective. When the Vietnam War lengthened and its cause and objective dimmed, America just quit.

Chapter 3

Facing the Storm

A few years ago I heard the following story.

A farmer who raised chickens found an abandoned eagle egg. Since the mother had been killed, the farmer took the egg and placed it under one of his setting hens. Eventually the eaglet hatched along with some peeps.

The farmer wanted the eagle to fit in, but its nature was too different. The eagle always walked alone, keeping its distance from the scratching chickens. As the eagle grew larger, the farmer clipped its wings so it would not fly away. But he could not clip the eagle's spirit. Day after day, while the chickens kept their beaks busy on the scraps in the barnyard, the eagle felt itself drawn upward.

Whenever a storm rolled over the area, the chickens ran to the barn but the eagle tried to stretch forth its wings and fly. It was useless, but anyone could see from its actions that this bird was no chicken.

Then one day came another great storm. Lightning streaked across the sky and thunder roared from miles around. The farmer was so busy with the oncoming storm that he didn't notice the eagle's feathers had grown back in. In the confusion, the eagle managed to climb atop a fence post as the chickens ran for cover.

Facing into the storm, the eagle felt a great sense of exhilaration as the wind blew against its feathers. Far up in the sky it spied another eagle, soaring high. Then a sharp cry pierced the air. Instinctively, the eagle stretched its wings and a sudden gust of wind carried it aloft. With a scream of victory the eagle took off into the air. Higher and higher it soared until it rode triumphantly above the storm.

I believe many Vietnam vets are like that eagle. Years ago we answered a call to leave the safety of America and face the storm in another country. We might not have known our full purpose for being there, but we knew there was a purpose.

When the war was over, we came back to the barnyard. We were told in one way or another that eagles were not welcome. Some of us had our wings clipped by anti-war protestors, others by family and friends, but most of us clipped our own wings. There was only one problem. We were no longer happy to be chickens. We had seen life and death and known the power that comes in offering oneself as a sacrifice for another.

Although we tried to conform, inwardly we were torn apart by our own hypocrisy. We wanted to reach out to other eagles, but we were afraid that they, too, had abandoned their high calling. Some of us even had heard God calling to us when we were in Vietnam, but at home He seemed far away.

Vietnam vets like myself, who pushed everything down inside, have paid a terrible price. We have hurt not only our own lives but also those of our families. Also, we have not contributed the benefit of our experience to the people in our communities who are trying to understand foreign affairs.

We needed to talk about what happened and America needed to listen to us. Instead, we let the storm over Vietnam cloud all the issues. We left the press and film makers with almost no one to oppose them as they told whatever distorted stories they selected. Even the ideal of fighting communism has become an embarrassment.

Vets need to soar again, not only for their own sakes, but also for the sake of the nation. Dangerous new storms are rising in America.

Communism Remains the Same

Ever since Mikhail Gorbachev launched the astounding reversal of Soviet repression, Americans have been rushing to embrace the Russian people. It has been a heartwarming, face-to-face reunion. As much as we need to love and welcome them, we must never forget that communist rulers can reverse their reforms at any moment. How many noticed that even while front page stories extolled the sailors' visits in Virginia, those newspapers also carried stories about Soviet spies?

In all the excitement, it is easy to forget what is wrong with communism. My generation is old enough to remember earlier flirtations with reform that were bitterly crushed: Hungary, 1956; Czechoslovakia, 1968; Solidarity, 1981.

We need to think about the Chinese students who touched the world with their bravery and their "Goddess of Democracy". We must not forget how the ruthless communist state mowed them down and removed all traces of their campaign for freedom. Communism is supposed to be a panacea for workers, but workers joined the students to protest its great failure. As NBC newsman John Chancellor said, "While its warlords and party bureaucrats grow fat, the Chinese People's Republic can't feed or house many of its people properly."

In the 1950s, the people of South Vietnam wanted freedom from the evils of communism just as much as the Chinese students wanted it in 1989. After the Vietnam War it became popular to say that the communistic North Vietnamese fought only because they were protecting their homeland against American aggressors. That was the justification of anti-war protestors, like actress Jane Fonda, who visited the enemy capital and condemned their own countrymen. This misconception has been costly for vets. It has kept them under a weight of false condemnation.

As the last tragic events in China's Tiananmin Square were unfolding, this report appeared in the **New York Times:**

> Desperate as they saw their friends fall and crimson stains spread on their chests, students and workers sought out foreign journalists and tugged them toward corpses.
>
> "We appeal to your country," a university student begged as bullets screamed overhead. "Our government is mad. There must be something that America can do."

Sorry, but America is no longer in the business of helping victims of communism, even with economic sanctions or statements of condemnation. "No more Vietnams" means that we no longer will respond to heart-rending cries. We feel sorry for you, but we soon will forget what you said. There is nothing we can do.

The Truth about the Villages

When we returned to America from Vietnam, we often were greeted by protestors shouting, "Baby killers!" Somehow they had the idea that our main occupation in Vietnam was to search out and destroy innocent children.

I remember what it was like to search those pitiful huts. It was necessary because of the type of guerilla warfare engaged in by our enemies. They forced their way into the villages of the South Vietnamese and used these simple, innocent people as a shield for their own protection. Far from hating us, many of the people welcomed us because they were terrified of the Viet Cong. The VC would stop at nothing.

I knew of Viet Cong who would attach a bomb to the back of a child and send him, unsuspecting, toward friendly American soldiers. They could care less that the child blew up along with the Americans.

We do not think like that in America. It was inconceivable to us that an adult could send an innocent child to his death. We always were looking for ways to help them, not harm them.

I never will forget the children I saw in one hut. They were probably two and three years old, but they all were naked. When I got closer, I discovered the reason. They were covered with rashes and sores. I felt so helpless, but I wanted to do something so I took a tube of ointment out of my pack and gave it to them. Then I scoured our supplies for anything else I could find that would help. There were too many physical needs for us to make much difference in the children's lives, but somehow we hoped that freedom would bring a change for the better.

Long before I arrived there, the Communists in Vietnam were committing atrocities. When Americans heard about those events, they felt that something must be done.

What was happening?

In 1954, according to the Geneva Accords, the North Vietnamese were required to permit the peaceful emigration of all who wished to leave. By that time, the Viet Minh were no longer an alliance of nationalistic groups but thoroughly communist.

Thousands rushed to take advantage of the opportunity to leave. They were willing to give up all they had ever known. The call of freedom was stronger than the call of their roots.

At that time, Dr. Tom Dooley, a Navy doctor who became a sort of folk hero for his work in Southeast Asia, was stationed at Haiphong, North Vietnam. His assignment was to provide humanitarian and medical attention in refugee camps for those leaving North Vietnam. A Roman Catholic, he considered such work for the U.S. government to be an expression of his faith.

During his time there, Dooley observed firsthand how communist rulers unify their people by "teaching" them how to think. The following is an example of what he saw.

> The Viet Minh aimed much of their propaganda at the children and teenagers of the nation, and they went to horrible lengths to make their propaganda stick. The first time I ever saw the results of a Communist "re-education" class was during the month of December.
>
> The Communists had set up their controls in the village of Haiphong. One day they visited the village schoolhouse and hauled seven children out of their class and

into the courtyard. All of them were ordered to sit on the ground, and their hands and arms were tied behind their backs. Next they brought out one of the young teachers with hands also tied. Now a new class began.

In a voice loud enough to reach the children who were still in the classroom, the Viet Minh accused their prisoners of treason. A "patriot" had informed the police that this teacher was holding classes secretly, at night, and that the subject of these classes was **religion**! They had even been teaching the catechism.

Because the seven had listened to the teachings of this instructor, the Viet Minh accused them of "conspiring against the state." As a punishment they were to be deprived of their hearing. Never again would they be able to listen to the teachings of evil men.

Two Viet Minh guards advanced on each child and one of them firmly grasped the head between his hands. The other then rammed a wooden chopstick into each ear. He jammed it in with all his force. The stick split the ear canal wide and tore the ear drum. The shrieking of the children was heard all over the village.

As for the teacher, he must be prevented from teaching again. Having been forced to witness the atrocity performed on his pupils, he endured an even more frightful one himself. One soldier held his head while another

> grasped the victim's tongue with a crude pair of pliers and pulled it far out. A third guard cut off the tip of the teacher's tongue with his bayonet. Blood spurted into the man's mouth and gushed down from his nostrils onto the ground. He could not scream: blood ran into his throat.
>
> Yet neither the teacher nor any of the pupils died.[1]

It is simply not true that America's only interests were imperialistic and economic. It is because Americans like Dooley saw these atrocities that they could not turn their backs on Vietnam when the French occupation ended. Those Americans saw what godless communism did to those whose only crime was a desire for freedom. Americans could not avert their eyes and walk on by–at least not until 1975.

During the course of the war Americans, too, committed atrocities, but with a major difference. The Americans' actions were considered crimes. Those deeds performed by the Communists were considered strategy.

Atrocities are not limited by nationality. They are not caused by one's race or national origin. They reveal the dark side of human nature. Communists and Americans who commit such actions have no fear of God or man. Atrocities destroy nations, not build them up. As Solomon wrote, "Righteousness exalts a nation, but sin is a disgrace to any people" (Prov. 14:34 NASB).

What Communists Believe

Ever since Soviet glasnost, Americans have been wondering why we were so afraid of the Soviet Union. The Russian sailors visiting in Norfolk, Virginia, seemed like such nice fellows. A headline in the local city newspaper read, "Soviet trip eliminates 'enemies,' Sailors wouldn't fight new friends." It is becoming increasingly difficult to recall why President Reagan ever considered the Soviet Union an "evil empire".

Regardless of how it may be clothed, communism is an evil system. Why? Consider the following reasons.

Karl Marx threw away all the centuries of established truth about who we are and how we arrived and rewrote the history of the human race. He claimed that the only idea worth fighting for was materialism–the eternal struggle between the classes to determine who would have the most power and possessions. Those who control the wealth, he said, always oppress their workers. Therefore, the workers must rise up and wrest control from their capitalistic oppressors.

Marx believed that all wars and revolutions were motivated by materialism. The only solution for ending these class struggles, he said, was communism. Under this system, after a temporary period where the leadership must rule with an iron hand for the good of everyone, the state would eventually wither away. In the communist utopia to come, the people no longer would need civil government. Everyone would voluntarily share all things. There would be no rich people and no poor people, only mass equality.

The logic of Marx and Engels sounded convincing to some, but there was one major problem. It didn't work. The "temporary period" of totalitarianism in the Soviet Union, for example, has lasted over seventy years. Countries like Cuba, Nicaragua and China, that followed the Marxist program, are in shambles. Marx had absolutely no understanding of human nature and was ignorant of the most basic facts of history.

I didn't know much of that in 1968 when I went to Vietnam. I just knew my country didn't want communism to spread and somehow my going there would help stop it. If I had read about communism even ten years ago and realized how important it was for us to halt it, I believe it would have prevented some of my personal struggles over the war.

There are several good reasons why communism is so destructive, and they are **not** all related to money.

The biggest problem with communism is its antagonism toward God. In America, our freedoms lasted all these years because our Founders established them on the foundation that God exists and that He has granted certain human rights no ruler can take away. The Declaration of Independence said, "We hold these truths to be self-evident, that all men are created equal, that they are endowed by their Creator with certain unalienable Rights, that among these are Life, Liberty and the pursuit of Happiness." Under communism, instead of acknowledging the rights that all men and women have as God's creation, the state usurps the role of the Creator of rights.

Whittaker Chambers, a former editor of **Time** magazine, made headlines about forty years ago when he admitted that he had been a member of the Communist Party and identified Algier Hiss, a highly placed official in several presidential administrations, as a fellow comrade. Although viciously accused of taking personal vengeance on Hiss and of trying to put himself in the spotlight, Chambers was not motivated by any of those things. He had discovered that the communist "faith" he had counted on to save the world was evil. He knew that if he said nothing it would destroy America.

During the Hiss trial, Chambers was constantly harassed by the press and by apologists for Hiss at the highest levels of government. Only his Christian faith, his family and the perseverance of the congressional investigation helped him survive. "Two faiths were on trial," Chambers said in his book **Witness**, "...two irreconcilable faiths of our time–Communism and Freedom."[2]

Chambers entitled his book **Witness** not because he was a witness against Hiss or even against communism. He was a witness **for** something. At great personal sacrifice he faced the storm and said, "Communism is wrong because something else is right."[3]

Communism fails in its mission to liberate mankind because no drive for freedom will ever succeed without God. Chambers wrote, "God alone is the inciter and guarantor of freedom."[4] Like the eagle drawn to the cry above it, we soar only when we are free.

Marxism not only puts man in place of God, it also puts the state in place of the family. Thus far, the state has been unable to conceive and bear children, but from birth a child becomes the property of the state. Marx said that was all in the child's best interests.

Marx wrote sarcastically to his critics, "Abolition of the family! Even the most radical flare up at this infamous proposal of the Communists."[5] But he protested that such was justified because parents could not be trusted to care for their children. Parental motives were always economic, he said, by how much work they could get out of their children. Therefore, the benevolent state must intervene in families to "stop the exploitation of children by their parents."[6]

Likewise, husbands could not be trusted to keep their wives. According to Marx, husbands were hypocrites, pretending to care for their wives but considering them as "prostitutes".

Because no God and no family was included in his ideal society, Marx could advocate the "intervention of society in education...to rescue education from the influence of the ruling class."[7] The state would teach all children that the world was in desperate straits and that its only hope was revolutionary change through communism.

Marx had no intention of limiting his re-education program to only one nation. The whole world must get involved. He wrote, "The working men have no country....United action, of the leading civilized countries at least, is one of the first conditions for the emancipation of the proletariat."[8]

American presidents knew about the international designs of Marxists and they wanted no part of the communist system. They did not believe what many of our children's textbooks now suggest—that there is little difference between our respective "values" and that Americans are just as imperialistic as the Soviets. These American presidents did not trust the Soviet overtures about peace because they knew what motivated these gestures. "While people are saying, 'Peace and safety,' " wrote the apostle Paul, "destruction will come on them suddenly" (1 Thess. 5:3 NIV).

Communism will never bring peace. It is based on a lie. Neither will communist leaders ever be our true friends. We do not have to hate them personally, but we must hate evil. Communism is evil. Beware lest you accept it as something good. The followers of its doctrines always have a plan to overthrow you. They will stop at nothing, and even pretend to work with you. Paul wrote that even satan can disguise himself as an angel of light (II Cor. 11:14).

In Vietnam the forces allied with Ho Chi Minh were willing to fight to the death because they thought they were saving their country. They had a promise of hope—a new society where no one would be in want and everyone would be free. Sure, this society would have to be accomplished by force. But if they would just make sacrifices for a short time, they would soon have heaven on earth.

Ho was so persuasive that his true followers never gave up. They continued to stream from North to South regardless of how many of them were wounded, killed or captured. They never lost heart at the number of lives lost or ruined, because theirs was a fight to the death. They had to change the world before it was too late.

Chambers said that it is very difficult for a deeply committed Communist to leave the party, because in doing so he believes he is abandoning all hope for the future of the world. Chambers himself left the Party only when he no longer could deaden his ears to the "screams" of those around the world whom the movement had destroyed. Before it was too late, he found something far better to put in its place.

In America we are fast losing the vision of true freedom for all mankind being something worthy of death. It is frightening to see American society beginning to resemble the Marxist model in state intervention of families and education. Most of us are just letting it happen because we don't know any better.

When I struggled with my own experience in Vietnam, I had to find answers. Were we right or were we wrong to be there? Did atrocities like the My Lai incident prove that we never should have been in Vietnam in the first place? If we were wrong, I knew I had to repent. But I discovered in my search that it was right for us to be there. It is something vets need to think about. If they continue to be double-minded about American involvement, they will continue to be in torment.

How We Can Face the Storm

It is time to face the storm instead of running from it. Vets need to say they are proud of serving in Vietnam. If they did anything wrong while there, they need to let the power of God cleanse them.

I believe there is a personal enemy, satan, who wants to keep us trapped in the past so that we fight the same battles over and over in our minds. Remember when we would take a hill, at great sacrifice, only to find out later that the Viet Cong had taken it right back? Those hills had to be retaken continually because the South Vietnamese did not do their job. In the same way, we continually will fight the same battles for our sanity if we do not maintain a stable lifestyle—emotionally, physically and spiritually.

Think about what it was like for you in Vietnam. Did the men in your unit commit one atrocity after another? Did they spend all their time trying to kill one another? Of course they didn't. Why have we allowed the American public to believe those lies? What has intimidated us?

I remember the first party I attended after I returned home. What a shock to find out that everyone was talking about America's evil involvement in Vietnam. I said nothing and from then on I hardly brought up the subject.

For all these years I avoided talking about Vietnam because I was afraid people would disagree with me. I have finally decided, "So what if they disagree?" We vets have something important to say.

We knew the cry of victory in 'Nam. We experienced the thrill of striving together for a common purpose. We risked our lives, our families and our futures to go to a foreign land and help a people about whom we knew almost nothing. Isn't that worth something?

I am not condemning those who stayed behind or escaped to Canada. That was twenty years ago. We should forgive and forget. We have had too many years of division. It is time to become united again. We need to understand the basis of freedom and share it with others.

We also need to guard against the subtle spread of Marxism in our own society. It is ironic that when communist countries are deteriorating on a worldwide scale, America's college professors, for example, continue to teach the superiority of Marxism.

My word to the vets is: Stand tall. Be proud. Because of our sacrifices, America continues to survive as a country. We shouldn't accept those judgements. We must stop saying that we were wrong and fought a totally unjust war. America made a lot of mistakes, but for a few years, at least, we helped the people in another country stop the spread of communism. Those mothers who lost their sons in the war did so for a just cause. As Jesus said, "Greater love hath no man than this, that a man lay down his life for his friends" (John 15:13).

Christian pacifists forget that Jesus Christ is the same yesterday, today and forever (Heb. 13:8). They need to read the Old Testament and see how Jesus is the Captain of the Hosts of Heaven, defending God's people.

America would be wrong to set out to conquer the world by force. But as our nation's Founders discovered, there comes a time when, having done all else that we can, we must rise to the occasion and refuse to hold back any longer.

The spirit of communism is a bewitching spirit. It lures its victims into submission and then attacks. The apostle Paul wrote, "You foolish Galatians! Who has bewitched you?" (Gal. 3:1 NIV). The word "bewitched" in the Greek is **baskaino**, meaning to fascinate by false representation, to malign.

In Vietnam we fought a physical enemy motivated by aggression. We took a stand and defended the country of our ally with strong military action. We also fought against principalities and powers of evil (Eph. 6:12).

When the vet fights depression, despair and a sense of futility, he fights the enemy of our souls, satan. Satan would love for us to never get victory in our lives because of the war. We must refuse to let him win. We must soar as the eagle.

The more I learn about the war and my place in it, the more I understand what a great spiritual battle I continue to fight. For too long a time I listened to the voices of defeat. Satan sets so many traps for us. We must be alert spiritually, mentally and physically to keep the victory.

The enemy would like us to remain silent about communism and about our understanding of right and wrong. So he intimidates us. He bombards our minds with our sins. In the Book of Revelation he is called the "accuser of our brethren" (Rev. 12:10). When we hear nothing in our minds but self-criticism, we never want to step out and be bold. We always feel like failures.

Thoughts like those pecked at my sore spots and made it almost impossible for me to succeed as a husband and as a father, let alone as a pastor. But I know who my enemy is now. I am not ignorant of his devices (II Cor. 2:11).

Instead of cringing or excusing myself when the enemy brings up my faults and failures, I am learning to agree with him. He is right. I do have faults and I have done things that were wrong, but I also have a great High Priest Who is faithful to forgive me and to cleanse me from all my unrighteousness (I John 1:9).

I refuse to cringe from any mention of the war just because I failed to do everything right. Sure, I made mistakes over there. None of us is perfect. What we as vets need to remember is that, in spite of our human weaknesses and the failings of our leaders, we still accomplished something important. For as long as we could, we said to the onslaught of communism, "This far and no farther."

End Notes

1. Thomas Dooley, **Doctor Tom Dooley, My Story** (Ariel Books, 1960), p. 42.

2. Whittaker Chambers, **Witness** (Henry Regnery Company, 1969), p. 4.

3. Ibid., p. 13.

4. Ibid., p. 16.

5. Karl Marx and Friedrich Engels, **The Communist Manifesto** (Penguin, 1967), p. 100.

6. Ibid., p. 100.

7. Ibid.

8. Ibid., p. 102.

Chapter 4

Effects of War

We were preparing to go out on an ambush. As night fell, we put on our camouflage and did our last minute checks with our weapons and gear. Seven of us were going about three hundred yards out from our perimeter. The mood was very tense. We knew there had been a lot of enemy activity the last few days. We had lost several men, even a few short-timers, who only had days to go before they went home.

We proceeded to go out on our ambush, notifying our lines that we were leaving, so they would know that any movement was us advancing to our position. Our job on an ambush was to go several hundred yards in front of our lines at night to surprise and catch the enemy off guard when they attacked our lines. It was important to leave after dark, so the enemy would not see us set up our position. We walked about five yards apart, staggering the formation so the enemy wouldn't catch us all together. Otherwise it would be easy for the enemy to frag us (throw grenades) and open fire.

On this particular night, we moved very slowly as the point man kept stopping to point out trip-wires and other possible enemy activity. I was next to the last person in line carrying an M-60 machine gun. Behind me was Roberts. I'll never forget Roberts. He wore these thick glasses (like coke bottles) and already had received three purple hearts. Once a soldier got three purple hearts he is supposed to go home, but Roberts volunteered to stay.

That night was very creepy. It was the kind where you can tell something is going to happen as you just feel the enemy all around. You can taste and smell the danger. It was a night when the adrenaline begins to flow and you know danger is very near.

Where's Roberts?

We began to move out and I turned to signal for Roberts to move. He was **gone**. No Roberts. I sent word up to the point that we had lost a man. Sometimes what the enemy would do, if he saw us going out on ambush, was grab the last man in line and slit his throat.

We continued to advance to our position about a hundred yards and set up our ambush; still no Roberts. We called back to our C.P. (command post) and reported what had happened.

Our captain told our squad leader to send two men back to try and find Roberts. Imagine it: two men going back toward our lines in pitch dark with the enemy all around. That was very dangerous, and it was asking a lot for two men to do.

Our squad leader told us what the captain said and asked for two volunteers. A good friend of mine, Lon, quickly said, "I'll go." Lon was one of those gung-ho type of guys, always daring. He was a tunnel-rat and always would walk point.

After he volunteered, there was this pause where no one said anything. I certainly was not going to volunteer. I had to stay with the M-60. That was my job. All of a sudden Lon says, "Tribus will go with me." "What?" I said, "What about the M-60?" Our dear squad leader quickly said he would stay with the gun as he knew how to fire it, if need be. "OK, give me a weapon," I replied. All that was available was a grenade launcher. It only carried one round.

Lon and I slowly started back toward our lines. Again the adrenaline flowed as everything inside us told us danger was ahead. Our own lines could open fire on us. We could get lost and have our own ambush hit us. The enemy lay waiting; and let's not forget Roberts. He could panic and open fire on us, if he were still alive.

The night played tricks on us, as we swore everything moved. Only our training and discipline kept us from shooting at everything we thought was moving.

This incident happened over twenty years ago, and I remember every detail as if it were yesterday.

Paralyzed by Fear

We continued through the jungle, looking for Roberts. Lon walked the point and I followed about five yards behind him. He would stop often, as he thought something moved, but then would continue, ever so slowly, ever so carefully. Each step could be our last one and we knew it.

Then Lon stopped for a long time. I walked up to him and asked what was wrong. "I can't move," he said. The adrenaline had flowed as everything intensified. He became unsure of himself and felt like everything was going to snap. "I've never been so scared in all my life," said Lon. I had to reach down inside myself for every ounce of strength I had, and said, "I'll take the point." I was just as terrified as Lon, but under that pressure something gave me that extra strength.

Suddenly the bush in front of us moved. We knew someone was there, and I called out, "Roberts." No answer. My reaction was to fire into the bush; but I thought I would advance ever so carefully. I walked right up to the bush and looked closer. These thick glasses looked back at me. I thought Roberts was dead. I reached into the bush and shook him. He began to gag and cough but he could not speak. He stood there paralyzed by fear, unable to catch his breath. The enemy had circled him and he had hidden in the bush.

Back Safe and Sound

After a few moments, we all gained back our strength and made our way to our ambush site, safe and sound.

Just a few days later, Lon was wounded seriously and sent back to the States.

That was just one episode of what happened to me twenty years ago in Vietnam. I remember how time and time again we had to react quickly and decisively. Under extreme pressure, our human bodies could do superhuman feats because of the rush of adrenaline.

One night we were guarding a bridge from the vantage of a gun tower. Rudy and Sonny were on guard in the tower as I slept on the ground. In the middle of the night the gun tower came crashing down with a mighty force. It had sand bags piled on its roof to protect us from enemy mortars. Sonny was somehow thrown free while Rudy was being crushed to death under the roof of the gun tower. Sonny grabbed the corner of the roof, and with one mighty pull lifted that roof with tons of sand bags upon it while Rudy crawled to safety. The next morning, Sonny, along with six other men, could not budge that roof one inch.

Effects of War

Every person who goes off to war realizes that lives depend upon him or her. Whether in combat or in supportive roles, we have intense pressure put upon us. Whether we actually go into combat or are on alert, depending upon every bit of training we have stirs up that life-saving emotion deep within us.

Our adrenal glands were made to produce adrenaline under extreme pressure or danger. However, whether in Vietnam, the Persian Gulf or any other war, these glands work more than usual. That is why war affects us emotionally, spiritually and physically.

When a person has dreams or flashbacks, that same adrenaline flows, producing the effect of actually being there. People under super amounts of stress will see these effects in their lives. It was true in the Vietnam War, and will be in the Persian Gulf War.

Look for the Signs

There are symptoms to look for in our lives. They are signs that show us something is wrong. If the "oil light" in your car blinks, it is a signal of something wrong. Just smashing out the light is not the answer. Here are a few signs to look for to see if the war has affected your life.

- Anger
- Anxiety
- Survivor's guilt
- Flashbacks
- Depression (more than usual)
- Withdrawal

- Nightmares
- No interest in family
- No interest in job
- Lack of memory
- Substance abuse
- Negative self-image
- Problems with intimate relationships

Keys for Recovery

It is possible for vets to leave these effects of war behind us. We can recover from that state of inner torment. The following are spiritual keys we need to use to unlock the doors that keep us locked out.

• **Repentance.** We must truly repent. With God, all things are possible (Mark 10:27). We must confess our sins as He is faithful and just to forgive us (I John 1:9). We must know that God understands and that the blood of Jesus can blot out that sin.

• **Trust.** Many of the Psalms teach us about basic trust in God. Many vets, because of being used, do not trust anyone. The Lord knows everything we have endured, even the things no one else understands.

• **Learn from your mistakes.** The Bible tells us that a righteous man falls seven times but he gets back up (Prov. 24:16). The enemy loves it when we make a mistake where he can throw it in our faces.

A news reporter asked Thomas Edison after he invented the light bulb, "How do you feel now being successful, after failing five thousand times?" Edison quickly replied, "I haven't failed five thousand times but succeeded five thousand times, in learning what doesn't work."

• **Spiritual warfare.** We must study the Word of God and let it work in our lives. An old wrestler once told me, "A good wrestler is never down, he's either up or he's getting up." Learn that we "wrestle not against flesh and blood, but against principalities, against powers, against the rulers of the darkness of this world, against spiritual wickedness in high places" (Eph. 6:12).

• **Prayer.** We must learn to personally spend time in prayer. It is important to take that time each day to pray to God and ask Him for help.

• **Forgiveness.** The key of forgiveness works both ways. We must learn to ask for forgiveness and learn to forgive. Forgiveness is an act of our wills; forgetting is a process. A lot of people feel God hasn't forgiven them because they still feel the pain. However, healing takes time. Believe God's Word that says He forgives us if we confess our sin to Him, and trust Him (I John 1:9). Many times we do not forgive even ourselves. Are we greater than God? If He forgives us, we should accept it and believe it, whether we feel forgiven or not.

• **Communication.** We must learn to communicate with those close to us and with others who have lived through similar circumstances. That will help us to not isolate ourselves and allow the devil to attack us. The devil goes after the weak lambs and devours them. God wants us in His fold for safety and for us to belong to Him.

• **Be under proper leadership.** God's government has laws and we must obey those laws. We need accountability in a place God has ordained. Seek God for His direction and read His Word. God says that if we ask for bread, He will not give us a stone (Matt. 7:9).

The Ambush of the Enemy

One of the first messages God gave me as a preacher was related to my military training. I was taught that, in jungle warfare, the enemy would wait to ambush us. Isn't that just the way it is? The devil waits until the last possible moment and then ambushes us. He tries to surprise us and hopes to catch us unaware.

When we were out on patrol the enemy would sometimes see us and set up an ambush. He would be very careful about springing the ambush because he wanted to be effective with his attack. For once he opened fire, he gave away his position. He wanted some key hits in the first rounds that he fired.

There were three men the enemy wanted to hit in his first burst of fire power. So he would study the platoon as we were on patrol and look for these three key men. First was the machine gunner. The reason the enemy wanted that man down quickly was often, after he opened fire, that gun would fire back at him. That M-60 could fire 560 rounds a minute with every fifth round a tracer, which zeroed in on the enemy. That is why in a fire-fight a machine gunner only lived about fifteen seconds.

I was a machine gunner. I was in over a hundred fire-fights and made it home because of the protection of God on my life. To me that speaks of our fire power of prayer. The enemy of our souls wants to destroy our prayer lives. Why? He knows the effect it has on the forces of darkness.

The second person the enemy wanted to kill in an ambush was the man carrying the radio on his back. He wanted to kill the man with the radio as soon as possible in order to destroy the communication for the platoon to any other allies. Once a fire-fight broke out, the radio-man called for air support and help from other units in that area.

In essence, the enemy of our souls wants to destroy our communication with others in the Body of Christ. **The devil hates unity.** He knows that if he can keep us isolated, we eventually will fall short of fulfilling God's purpose in our lives. The devil wants us divided. He uses gossip, jealousies, hatred, strife, envyings, etc. We must learn that we need each other in the Body of Christ and that churches need other churches. We have to keep those lines of communication open. For if one can put a thousand to flight, two can put ten thousand to flight (Deut. 32:30). We can accomplish **more** together than we can divided. We never know when we will need each other, so we must keep those lines open and ready.

The third man the enemy wanted down right away in an ambush is the **leader.** The enemy knew that if he could kill the leader with his first blast of fire power, the team then would be confused and **easy pickings.** Out in the jungle, the leaders did not wear any special medals or signs of authority. They just fit in with all the others.

Isn't it ironic that Judas had to kiss Jesus to point Him out? He looked like everyone else. He didn't have any special dress or medals of authority.

We need leaders in the church who have authority from God, who are not in the ministry for themselves. We need leaders who are servants, willing to be with the people of God.

In recent years we have seen leaders be attacked by the fire power of the enemy. They have been ambushed. We need to learn the tactics of the enemy and be ready for his ambush. Leaders must keep themselves clean. Jesus said that satan came and found nothing in Him (John 14:30). That is to say, the devil came and could find nothing in Jesus to which he could claim rights.

The enemy has attacked the leadership for years. He will continue to do so as it keeps the troops from doing their jobs. The enemy wants to destroy any leadership that is of God, whether it be in the home, government or church. He hates

God's government and God's authority and sets traps and ambushes. But the apostle Paul tells us that we are not ignorant of the devil's devices (II Cor. 2:11).

We must be on guard continually and fight the good fight of faith. A good soldier constantly trains and stays alert physically, mentally and emotionally. May we ever be so mindful to keep alert in the spirit, stay prayed up and careful to watch for the ambushes of the enemy. May we learn to assault the ambush the enemy would set and send him running.

Chapter 5

Where's the Band?

I still remember the day I left Vietnam. I was on ship when I said good-bye to a lot of my friends. Sonny and Rudy were in a hospital somewhere and Ted had gone home a few months earlier. As I left I felt sort of bad because I could leave but they had to stay. Some would make it, some would die. Others would never be the same again.

But I finally was on my way home. I couldn't believe it. I really did think I would die in Vietnam. Three hundred ninety-five days came down to one. It seemed like an eternity. So much had happened. I saw more in those thirteen months than I had seen in my entire life of eighteen years. I thought I aged about ten years, mentally and emotionally. I certainly had a good look at the world and at a side of it that would have an impact on me for the rest of my life. I didn't know that at the time though, because I held everything inside. I really did not trust anyone.

Our plane took off from Vietnam to Okinawa, where we spent three days. I felt numb. It was as though it were all a dream. What a difference from when I joined the service. Everyone was so polite and grateful for who we were. I felt so proud.

Little did I know that in a few days, in the old USA, people would not be so receptive. I could not figure out what they thought. Some wanted to be nice, but no one really wanted to talk about the war. I later could see people wondering what I was like or if something had happened to me. Things changed so much in that one year. Many did not even care. Not that anyone could blame them, they just were so busy with college or work.

The Plane Trip

Finally the day came for us to leave Okinawa and begin our journey halfway around the world, with a stop in Hawaii. We would be in the air about eleven hours, so there must have been plenty of fuel on the plane. It was a very large plane and as we all boarded there was a quietness about the whole process. Here were hundreds of soldiers who were in Vietnam and I did not know one of them; however, we all shared the same thoughts.

Then the moment arrived: Prepare for takeoff. The giant plane raced down the runway and as it left the ground and became airborne the entire group of soldiers, from all over Vietnam, began to clap and shout in one accord. What a rush of energy and joy as we began to climb higher. All I could think of was that the next stop would be somewhere "safe".

As the plane continued to climb, the captain began putting the landing gear up and we could feel the hum.... Then we heard and felt something jam. Everyone became totally silent. This same group, who with one voice shouted and celebrated in knowing they were finally headed home, in the same unity became suddenly silent. We all could sense that something was wrong.

After a very long minute the captain came on the speaker and said that the landing gear jammed halfway and he could not get it up or down. We circled a few times and then he said that we would have to land the plane because he could not fly across the ocean with the landing gear stuck. But before we could land, we had to fly out over the ocean and dump all the fuel. About an hour went by as we all watched the fuel pour from the plane into the Pacific Ocean. I would never forget my thoughts at that time, because all I thought was, "I made it through 395 days in Vietnam as a machine gunner and now I am going to be killed in a plane crash going home."

We prepared for a crash landing. As we approached the runway my heart pumped like crazy. The palms of my hands were sweating as I rubbed them together, praying as fervently as when I was in the bottom of a foxhole with mortars going off all around and bullets coming so close I could hear them whistling by my head. Closer and closer, lower and lower the plane came to the runway. Then with a great jolt the plane touched the ground and coasted to a stop. All were safe. No one was hurt; we made a safe landing.

I didn't know how much more I could stand. My head was splitting; there was so much tension. Then we had to get off the plane and on to another. We had to do it all over again. This time when we left the ground, there was no shouting, no clapping, no excitement. All we thought was, "Get us home."

We landed in Hawaii for a few hours to refuel and then flew to California. I was in California for three days before flying to Pennsylvania. It was a very strange experience when we landed at my hometown. Just a few days before I was in the rice paddies of Vietnam and that night I would be eating supper with my family.

My mother, sister and uncle met me there. I was the only soldier on the plane and no one seemed to notice. I was very quiet and really did not know what to expect. I guess if it had been World War I or World War II a host of people would have met us as a unit coming home. There would have been a lot of excitement and joy with everyone coming home at one time. Oh, I was happy I was home, but something seemed to be missing. Where's the band?

As I sat in our living room that night, I could not help thinking of my buddies in Vietnam. It wasn't fair that I was home and they were still there. I had thought at one time, "How could anyone go home from 'Nam and then volunteer to come back?" But now those thoughts began to go through my mind. I actually began to think that I might want to go back.

Little did I know what I would go through in the next few years. At night I couldn't sleep. I could not stand being among a group of people. I preferred to eat alone, and was very jumpy if anyone came up behind me. It was nothing for me to go out and get drunk. I felt so bad one night when I punched one of my good friends right in the mouth as he tried to stop me from fighting someone else. The very next day I went to his house and apologized to him. He could not understand what was wrong with me. As a matter of fact, I myself did not know. I really was messed up. I did not know what I wanted. I would find myself crying for no reason, just feeling very low.

It wasn't long afterwards that I got saved and asked Christ into my heart. I kept very busy in the Lord and within a year married and went to Bible school. I felt I was fulfilling the will of God in my life, but I still fought the war in my mind. I would dream about being in Vietnam, then wake up sweating and fearful. When I dreamt about it, the same feelings would be there: great tension, with pressure from all around and from within.

That was key, "within". These things were within me. I could feel the pressure in my spirit. I prayed, asking the Lord to help, and He is faithful to help in time of need. Still, I had to see that the problem was in my spirit. Many preachers believe that once a person is saved, he or she is healed of all these things. However, I needed a healing in my spirit; in my soul. Christ did come into my heart and I did become a new creature. But I needed to deal with the old self. I tried to tell myself that these things were not happening, but I was putting a Band-Aid on cancer. It was a root worked down into my spirit that now had to be rooted out by the Word of God. It couldn't be cast out. It was not a devil, but a root of bitterness. A root of confusion. A root of resentment. I covered it up as best I could, but it was there. To see all I saw in Vietnam and to experience all I experienced became a part of me.

Paul says in Second Corinthians 7:5 that he fought battles within and without. I was fighting this battle within me while outwardly I as a vet battled the anti-war movement. No one seemed to care. Nothing seemed to be enough. It seemed like no one understood what was happening to the Vietnam vet. Where was the appreciation? In later years when some appreciation finally did come, the vets cried, "Too little, too late."

I want to share a little story that helped me a lot. I heard it about ten years ago and I let it sink into my spirit to help me uproot the thoughts of no one caring. It may not seem important, but give the story some thought. I know that vets know what I'm talking about. But let it sink into your spirit. Don't just read it, really believe and know it to be the Word of the Lord.

A missionary was coming home by ship from a long trip. He had been ministering the Word of the Lord to a foreign people and was very weary. He had been gone for several years. He had lived without the comforts of home, out in the bush in a hut with native people. When it came time for him to go back home, he could not even afford to fly. Instead he took a ship on a very long voyage because the cost was cheaper. For those years that he was gone he had poured out his life.

As the ship pulled into port he noticed a great crowd of people. Great excitement was in the air. A band was playing, and the place was electrified. He could not believe it, there was so much joy and people yelling and singing. As the ship pulled closer and came to a stop, he realized the band was not playing for him but for some celebrity who was also on board. The missionary watched as people rushed to this other person. The people had so much joy to see the famous man and be close to him. The missionary couldn't help but feel depressed as the crowd moved with the celebrity and everything became very quiet.

Very humbly he picked up his luggage and looked for someone to meet him. No one came. He was there alone. So he took a cab and went to a small hotel. He checked in and, completely exhausted, fell across the bed. He could not hold back the tears. As he wept he simply asked the Lord how a man who was famous could get such a homecoming. "It's not fair," he said, "here I was doing the work of the Lord all these years, and when I come home, **nothing.** No one to meet me. No cheering. No band." Then a still small voice whispered to him. It was the voice of God, and He so tenderly said, "Son, you're not Home yet."

We need to realize that our reward is coming. There is going to be a homecoming like we've never imagined. Jesus will have the best band and the best celebration that we could ever devise. Eye has not seen what the Lord has prepared for us. Let this thought stick with us and in our spirits, that the Lord will reward those who have been faithful. When people get their rewards here, from other people, they are only temporary. God's reward is eternal.

Chapter 6

Healing the Wounds

In every war there are casualties; physically, emotionally and spiritually. Those who are wounded physically need time to heal, as they are tended by doctors and the medical personnel. The same holds true for those wounded emotionally and spiritually. Why do we expect everything to heal instantly? For some the healing process is longer and more difficult than for others, as we cannot see the depth of the inner wound.

Many of the Persian Gulf vets soon will find that life does not pick up where it left off. We cannot separate families for months at a time, and expect everything to be the same afterwards. The enemy of our souls has been busy at work as he saw men and women going off to war and the home suffering through that intense time. As these vets return home, we enjoy great victory and much celebration; however, we must realize that wounds may surface after the little honeymoon is over. Many hope and pray for no after-effects, but already we are seeing problems. Someone can bleed inside spiritually or emotionally while we are blinded to what is happening.

Life Is in the Blood

There is a story in the Bible in Matthew 9:20-22 where Jesus healed a woman with an issue of blood. Twelve years she sought for help, spending all her money in her search for health.

From the Mosaic law we learn that anyone with an issue of blood is unclean. Even a man with a running issue is unclean. Now remember, not only is that person unclean, but anyone he or she comes in contact with, is unclean. The Word of the Lord also teaches us that the life is in the blood; therefore, people who bleed are seeing their very life drained out of them. So as we look at this woman in Matthew 9:20-22, we see that she has a very limited relationship with her family, has no friends, is weak physically and is drained emotionally, spiritually and financially. Now we begin to see a little deeper into what really happened.

Jesus came walking by, and this woman, in desperation, pressed through the crowd and touched the hem of His garment. Jesus stopped and asked, "Who touched me?" Can you imagine, with thousands of people around Him, that He would ask such a question? But something had happened in the spirit, that no one physically saw.

I can see that woman knowing that something had happened to her. For the first time in twelve years she felt such a rush of life and strength because this issue became clean in her life. Within her own mind there was an emotional release, to know she would have a full relationship with her husband and could embrace her children. Oh, what a moment of great joy she experienced because she pressed through to touch Jesus, the great Healer. No one else in the crowd realized that anything had happened.

Perhaps you have an issue that is draining the very life out of you. It affects not only you, but also others with whom you come in contact. For years I did not realize that someone could hemorrhage internally and die. You cannot see any external bleeding. Now, spiritually, you can die from an issue in your life that is draining you spiritually and emotionally. You need to be healed. Only Jesus can heal that wound. You must press through the circumstances of life to touch Jesus and have His power released into your spirit. You will never be the same. You have lived with that issue long enough; it has cost you time and energy and affected others around you. It is time to press through.

Jesus Is Passing By

Now is the time to make up your mind to do something about your life and about the issues in your life. If you feel that energy being drained from your life, and you know deep within your own heart that you need healing, then now is the time. If you feel that no one cares or sees the death you are dying, it's time. It's time for **you** to make that move, and press through every thought, every obstacle and every spiritual enemy and touch Jesus. He is there to release His power into your spirit and into your life. It is not a time for self-pity and for expecting everyone to come running to you. Jesus doesn't make an issue of your problem; why should we? Remember, we don't see the wounds deep within your mind and in your spirit. But Jesus sees, and He waits for you to do something about it. Now is your time; press through.

Chapter 7

Christians Are Not Exempt

In the first chapter I related how my good buddy Sonny called. I had no time for him because I was busy doing the work of the Lord, or so I thought. About five years later I found myself fighting a battle for which I was unprepared. I thought I had everything together; you know, family and ministry doing well. However, little did I know that some things were buried deep inside me.

The average age of the soldier in Vietnam was 19; now he is between 40 and 50. I had heard something about mid-life but never expected it could have anything to do with me. After all, I was an ordained minister. I was saved in 1970 and really gave my heart to the Lord. All seemed okay on the outside, but inside some things were not going so well. I found myself withdrawing from people and letting some things slip in my walk with the Lord. I didn't pray as much and became less involved with the work of God.

Swallow that Pride

I did not understand what was happening inside me, yet I still counseled others on how to deal with their problems. I felt like such a hypocrite, yet to whom could I tell what was happening? Tension was building in my home as my wife and I would argue. The kids, Michael and Michele, were very much aware that something was wrong. But what to do? My wife, Joanne, called some of our minister friends to ask for prayer. Everyone wanted to help, but this war kept raging inside me.

One day I decided to try to visit my buddy Sonny. I don't know what I expected but I felt I had to do something. I remembered that he lived around San Antonio, Texas, and bought a ticket to go there. I never told my wife I hadn't called him. I just felt I had to go.

I talked to a few other vets who told me that they had tried to look up some old buddies and were very disappointed. One vet told me that he had saved a guy's life and when he called this guy, the man said he didn't want to see him. I took all that into consideration, but I still had to take the chance. If Sonny rejected me, I was prepared. So off to Texas I went. At the time Joanne and the kids didn't know what was going on, but Joanne told me later that she trusted God to keep me. She knew that something was deeply wrong and I had shut her out, but she prayed and trusted God for me.

When I arrived in Texas I located Sonny's number. He had moved about an hour away from where I was. Now it all came down to a phone call. I was nervous inside and had to swallow some pride, but I made myself pick up the phone.

I called the number and heard that big Texan voice answer. "Sonny here," he said.

I answered, "Sonny, this is Paul Tribus."

"Hey, buddy," he replied, "what you need?"

"Well, I'm here in San Antonio and sure would like to see you."

"That's great!" he said, and told me he would drive down the next day to pick me up. He would take the day off to spend with me.

The next day I waited for him to pick me up. I was really excited. We knew a lot about each other. After all, we had spent months together, out in the bush, with no TV. Over there we had plenty of time to talk and to share as we faced death every day.

The knock came at the door and there stood my good friend. We talked for a few minutes and I asked him to forgive me for the way I had treated him when he had called a few years ago. There were no hard feelings and we shared, talked and remembered old times. Then we called Rudy in Lyford, Texas, and he was so thrilled that we called. Rudy and Sonny were both wounded just shortly after I left the bush.

So, for two days we had a great time and I felt something good inside me. I believe I was searching for something lost somewhere inside me.

My family was glad when I came home. They wanted so much to help, but it was difficult for them to understand. I was so thankful for a wife who understood enough to trust God in this situation.

Yet I knew something was still wrong deep inside me. Seeing my old buddy was a big help and it fulfilled some of the emotional needs. But this war kept raging.

Mid-life? Maybe I was facing it head on. But I'm a Christian!

No Substitutes

This part of my life is hard to discuss because people always want to tell the bright side of victory. The next few years were anything but victorious for me. I had prided myself on the strength I had in the Lord for years. Now I was falling apart. I even went to a doctor and cried because I was so emotionally upset. She put me on pills to help me relax. I wound up taking them too often and found myself hooked. I would count the pills in the bottle because I was scared that they might run out.

I thought I literally was going out of my mind. I would cry all the time and felt this tremendous pull in a battle for my mind and my soul. I wasn't right and I knew it. I was lying to my wife about the pills. She thought I quit taking them. To avoid an argument, I would just lie. I thought I was doing the lesser of two evils. Oh, how the enemy tricks us and we become deceived!

I tried for months to quit those pills, but it just got worse. "I'm a Christian," I cried, "an overcomer." I prayed, cried and rebuked those things. Nothing happened until I really determined in my heart, "I am the Lord's." Then one day I just quit. What I couldn't do before, just happened. I believe people were praying for me, and God in His love had mercy on me.

I am not proud of what happened but it worked something into me. I found myself being more tender toward people who are weak toward vets and even toward things I don't understand.

The devil is real, and I actually thought I was exempt from any such attack. God wanted to clear something inside me—pride. Now I try to stay humble before the Lord. That means to be no better or no worse than anyone else.

It is a constant battle, but with prayer, our families and the people of God, we can make it.

Chapter 8

The Gulf War Is No Exception

Suppose someone rapes your little sister, then proceeds to take over the family business through force. Do you ignore it? Do you hope someone else will take the responsibility? Or does there come a time when you must take action, even at the risk of your own life?

America has come to help in many situations like those. Throughout history we have seen different men arise with the spirit of anti-Christ. From the Bible we see men such as Nimrod, Nebuchadnezzar and Herod. In more recent times, men such as Hitler, Ho Chi Minh and Saddam Hussein have arisen. We find it hard to believe that these men actually thought they could rule unless we know the Bible and realize they are possessed by the devil himself. In First John 2:18, John tells us that there are many anti-Christs, or many with the spirit of anti-Christ.

Is It Right to Go to War?

We are blessed to live in America, which never has sought to conquer or rule the world through force. Sure, we have laws and rules to live by, but by the same token, we are not the aggressor. However, when we must defend our country or help another, a time may come for war. Ecclesiastes 3:1 tells us, "To every thing there is a season, and a time to every purpose under the heaven." Verse eight says, "A time to love, and a time to hate; a time of war, and a time of peace." No one should want to go to war; it is a dreadful thing. But there comes a time when it must be.

People say, "Hindsight is 20-20." Looking back to the Vietnam War twenty years ago, my conclusion is that we did not lose the war militarily, but politically. That is why Vietnam has been mentioned so much in conjunction with the war in the Gulf. We need to learn some lessons from Vietnam, both physical and spiritual ones. It must be known that we cannot take individuals into a war and expect them to be the same. War will definitely change them, and it will affect them both now and later. (We dealt with the war that rages on in the first chapter.) For years afterwards men and women must deal with split second decisions they made under stressful situations.

Again, looking back over my own life and experiences in war, I would not want to go and do it again, but I would not trade the experience I have gained.

Is the War in the Gulf Like Vietnam?

Twenty years ago I heard a man say that he did not believe in war. In fact, he was a strong opponent of the war and protested whenever he could to show his opinion. A Vietnam vet friend of mine told this man that he went over to fight to be sure he always will have that right. It's strange, but I heard the same thing said between two people concerning the Persian Gulf War.

A lot of people ask the question, "Is the Persian Gulf War like Vietnam?" Now please don't mistake us when we say that we don't want another Vietnam. It is in the respect that people do not want another long, drawn out war which seems to go on forever. Vietnam lasted sixteen years. That is why people get upset when these two wars are compared. However, to answer our original question about the war in the Gulf being like the war in Vietnam: Absolutely. They are both wars.

War and Memory

When the war in the Gulf was announced, a lot of Vietnam veterans began to have problems. Why? I myself triggered a lot of old memories as I watched television. Out there in the battlefield you put things into your mind and into your spirit that, unless the Lord Jesus helps you and you look to Him for that help, cause flashbacks and trigger those old feelings.

Let me explain further. Suppose when you were a child your father became very upset with you. You were home alone watching a scary movie on a rainy night. The phone rang and it was someone telling you bad thoughts. You hang up the phone and get really scared. You run to the door to make sure it was locked. About the time you reach for the lock the door flies open. You stand there petrified, and let out a scream. It is your father, and now you've annoyed him. He becomes very angry. You try to tell him what happened, but he does not understand and in his anger smashes the lamp on the coffee table.

Now, let's suppose years later you are at home alone and it is raining. You switch on the television and there is that same scary movie. Coincidentally, the telephone rings, and it triggers all these old feelings of your past. The adrenaline starts to flow and for that moment you remember every feeling you had years ago because of that previous intense moment.

Now you can imagine what veterans go through when through the course of the day things happen that trigger these actual feelings that go back years in their pasts. These men and women, both in Vietnam and the Persian Gulf, were in life and death situations every day. Even on calm and quiet days, when we thought nothing was going to happen, we would suddenly be attacked. We learned to be on guard at all times.

I heard of a man, once in combat in Vietnam, who twenty years later found himself becoming very depressed and feeling some of the old anger. As some of his fellow vets reached out to him in prayer and understanding, they realized that he seemed to be getting these feelings every Friday. After looking into the matter a little more closely, they found out that Friday was garbage day. You might think, "What does that have to do with his feelings?" But it was discovered also that he helped to bring back our own dead soldiers in body bags. Years later, coming home from work, the street would be lined with garbage bags. Those plastic bags triggered these feelings, especially on dreary, rainy days.

We thought PTSD (Post Traumatic Stress Disorder) was only for the Vietnam vet, but all we did was give it a name. Vets of every war have had its symptoms, such as tension, isolation, depression, guilt, denial, etc. That includes the Persian Gulf vet.

The Role of Adrenaline

Probably as you read this book you can recall some instance in your life that was very intense, when your adrenaline started pumping. From time to time you can remember every detail, even down to a smell, of those moments. I have seen people do things with supernatural strength when the adrenaline started to flow. It is such a rush of the body to protect itself from harm.

This rush of adrenaline is one of the main problems of being in a war zone. Your body has adrenal glands which are small glands attached to the kidney. They secrete adrenaline in cases of extreme fear or in life-threatening situations. The problem with them in war is that they are used so much. We have no control over it; it is a normal body reaction. However, in normal life these glands may secrete once every few weeks, perhaps in a close call with a car, or from seeing someone else in a life and death situation. In war they can secrete several times a day, that without your knowing it, wears down the body physically and emotionally.

I have learned from my own life that things I saw and experienced twenty years ago still can be triggered. The mind is an incredible thing. It takes pictures and stores them, without your even realizing it did so. Did you ever dream about someone you haven't seen or thought about in years? Possibly something during the day triggered a thought that retrieved the picture from the back of your mind.

A short time ago I was out for breakfast and somehow wound up eating steak and eggs. Now I usually do not order steak and eggs. In fact, I never order it. I like to eat eggs and toast. When the order came, it triggered a thought deep within me that went back over twenty years.

While in Vietnam, we would go on ship every month or so, as I was with a floating battalion. We would go on ship for a few days and then go from ship to hot areas. We would make beach landings from boats or be flown by helicopter into areas where there was a lot of enemy activity, or where another unit in a lot of trouble needed help.

I used to love to go aboard ship. It would ensure for us a night's sleep without bugs, snakes or enemy ambushes. I still could remember the knot in my stomach, sleeping in the bush and always being on alert. There was always such fear, of not knowing what was going to happen. At any time an ambush may hit or a booby trap go off, and in one split second change your whole life.

Oh, but on ship we had a short rest from all of that. Every time our Marine unit boarded the ship, those sailors treated us like royalty. They made sure we were well taken care of for the time we would be aboard.

Now every time we prepared to leave the ship, the opposite feelings would occur. We knew we were going back into the battle as we cleaned our weapons, made sure we had enough ammunition and saddled up for the journey; knowing deep in our hearts that some of us would not make it back. I think that is the reason those sailors treated us so nicely; they knew we were fighting a severe war on ground, as they supported us with guns from ships. We all worked together.

However, every time we were going on an operation and preparing to leave ship, that morning the navy always would cook for us, (you guessed it), steak and eggs. It was called our victory breakfast. After a few times I had mixed emotions when we ate our victory breakfast, knowing of the battle waiting for us and of the friends we would lose. Many times as I ate that breakfast, sometimes dressed with my battle gear, I would bow my head and try with all my heart to be thankful and to look at the bright side for that moment.

Now you can imagine how I felt some twenty years later out for breakfast with a few friends, when the order for everyone was steak and eggs. It triggered all those old memories. In just a few seconds I saw the faces of some of the men with whom I served. Some are still alive, some were killed. I remembered the sailors and the smell of that steak and those eggs just as if I had gone back twenty years. Oh, what a rush I had in my emotions and my thoughts, and here I was with friends trying to enjoy a simple meal.

But I've learned some things over the years, so I simply told God what it meant to me. We bowed our heads and gave a special thanks to God for the meal and for His blessing in our lives. Without letting the others know, I told the Lord that it still hurt deep inside and that I was offering it to Him. I told Him that I still hurt for the men that I had served with, and for the times I felt I was wronged, cheated and used. Then I raised my head and enjoyed my victory breakfast.

On the Homefront

Now remember, as the storm clears in the Mid-East we must be prepared to deal with the homefront. Families all over this country are hurting because we had to send men and women off to war. Twenty years ago, as Vietnam vets returned home, they were torn to see what was happening on the homefront. America was split over the war issue, as we lost our vision for being there.

When I went to Vietnam I was not aware of the spiritual warfare I was getting into there. Years later we learned that while we were in Vietnam, Buddhist monks prayed a three-fold curse on any American who fought in the war. They prayed that 1.) we would find no peace; 2.) we would be angry men; and 3.) we would be wanderers for the rest of our lives. I have seen, in my own experience, how these evil spirits affected my life and the lives of many veterans. As I and others dealt with many veterans, we prayed and bound those spirits in the mighty name of Jesus. We have seen men set free from years of torment.

We must learn how to wage spiritual warfare for those who come home from war. Once any war is ended, many bring it home with them. Only the peace of God can bring healing to the spirits and souls of those tormented by the effects of war.

There must be total cooperation in the home, to pull together, as the healing power of God flows. Remember, family, these warriors coming home bring back memories that have put a deep mark on their minds and spirits. It takes time and prayer as God heals the wounds the devil has inflicted on the veterans of war.

Ephesians 6:11 tells us, "put on the whole armour of God, that ye may be able to stand against the wiles of the devil." Verse sixteen tells us to take "the shield of faith, wherewith ye shall be able to quench all the fiery darts of the wicked." When the apostle Paul wrote this passage, he knew what the Roman army used for warfare and likened that to spiritual warfare. He tells us to take the sword of the spirit, which is the Word of God (v. 17). He likened that sword to the Word.

Now consider this shield of faith. Paul saw many times what the Roman army would do. Can you imagine a platoon of soldiers walking down a street? There are five rows, and about twenty soldiers in a row. They all have a shield to protect them individually, but now they move as a unit. The five in front hold their shields straight ahead. The row on the left all hold their shields to the left. The row on the right all hold their shields to the right. All the others hold their shields over their heads; thus forming a human tank that walks against the darts of the enemy.

The family must form such a unit to fight against the fiery darts of the wicked one. If one of us tries to fight alone, it is a lot easier for one of those darts to reach us, but together we can win the battle.

The enemy has stolen months and years from those who went to war. But God has promised to restore the years that the enemy has stolen, as we yield to His Word and look to Jesus. Man can work only from the outside in, but Jesus works from the inside out. We have seen hundreds of vets come to Jesus, seen them be healed body, soul and spirit. It takes a lot of prayer, love, understanding and patience as we turn to God for the answers. If we run to the world for answers, we will get worldly answers; but if we turn to God and to His Word, then we will receive godly answers.

Chapter 9

After the Storm

As with any storm, there must be a clean-up afterwards. The same holds true with any war. Not only is there a reconstruction of cities and towns; there also must be a restoration of lives and a time of pulling together.

I believe now is a time for pulling together more than ever before. Vets must reach out to vets. We who went through the Vietnam War came home rejected and wounded. Some have likened us to abused children. Our country turned its back on us and the church was unprepared with answers or help. Everyone just hoped it would all be better if we just went on.

If a child is abused, he or she doesn't wish all children to be abused. Now is the time for those who have faced war and know the power of God in their lives to reach out to our younger brothers and sisters.

Two People in Quicksand

In order to help someone else, we first must know the power of healing in our own spirits and have met our own needs with Jesus and the Word of God. Just understanding problems is not enough. We must be established in the Word of God. Many people are attending "spiritual warfare seminars," but they need an encounter with God. Two people in quicksand cannot help each other. One of them must be on a rock. It is not enough to just have knowledge; we should know the answer. The answer is in having the reality of Jesus Christ in our individual lives.

The Storm Settles

My wife and I were in the flood of 1972 in Pennsylvania. After the flood waters receded and the storm ceased, it left a lot of destruction. If we had just looked at the damage, we would have asked ourselves if we would ever get the job done. It took a lot of work, time, energy and equipment. But restoration came.

You may look at your life and feel there is no hope, but God is waiting.

During the war in the Gulf we saw churches and prayer meetings all over the country. Many cried, "No more Vietnams!" We have learned from our mistakes. Twenty years ago the church was unprepared, but not this time. All over the country, special church services were held and people rallied to support our troops.

Now as life gets back to normal and the storm settles, we begin to see a little clearer. We have a lot of work to do. We need to roll up our spiritual sleeves and get to work. But remember that the devil is not going to quit. We must apply the principles presented in the previous chapters of this book to continue steadfast in the faith.

The Anointing Breaks the Yoke

God desires to heal you, body, soul and spirit. Jesus is a healer. He wants you to know that He desires you to prosper and be strong. People concentrate on the outside, while God starts from the inside. Many get caught up in physical health, but God wants to heal your spirit.

People feel that something will hit them and break the yokes and bondages in their lives. Many go to every prayer line, yet still live very unfruitful lives. They want everything instantly. But when a farmer puts a yoke on a young ox, that yoke is eventually broken, not from without but from within. As he grows, eats and gets stronger every day the yoke is broken.

That is why the anointing we have is within. It is important for us to eat the Word, grow in God and grow stronger every day. Then we can watch those yokes be broken in our lives! This book is not intended to give the illusion that everything is instant. Rather, it gives keys and principles that will work. We must learn to do things God's way, as our ways will always lead us into more problems.

No Victory without Battle

Listen to the words of Theodore Roosevelt.

> The credit belongs to the man who is actually in the arena, who's face is marred by dust and sweat and blood, who strives valiantly; who errs and comes short again and again, who knows the great enthusiasms, the great devotions, and spends himself in a worthy cause, who at the best knows the triumph of high achievement and who, at the worst, if he fails at least fails while daring greatly, so that his place shall never be with those cold and timid souls who know neither victory nor defeat.

Oh, how these words speak to our souls. Never is there a victory unless there is a battle. The greater the battle, the greater the victory. But we must let the Lord open our spiritual eyes.

War has affected many, many lives. It affects not only the life of the person who fought, but also of family, friends and all whom his or her life will touch. This book is not for the vet only, but for the many who became casualties along the way.

May you reach out to the Lord and fulfill the purposes of God in your life, whole and strong, as a good soldier of Jesus Christ. Endure the battles of life and know that victory is at hand!

Chapter 10

Moving Forward

We have learned how we need to be healed and begin our recovery. Along the way we may suffer some setbacks but we must continue the fight of the faith. We all need to find our places in life and seek the Lord's will for our lives.

Some are well on the road to recovery while others need to take the first step. My prayer for you is that this book will help you along the road. You may be a casualty of war or of someone wounded on the homefront. All over the nation, families are hurting, not knowing what happened. Either way, you've let the enemy ambush you and now you need to re-group, become strong and assault that ambush.

Part of the healing process is to help others. I know that is difficult, but one of the things the Lord wants you to do is to give. In your need, you must learn to pour out. You can be a blessing to others who are hurting. Too often we all find ourselves being so self-centered. Always seeking our own rights and our own ways only brings earthly satisfaction.

Ask God to help you look around you, upward and outward. In helping others you are blessed with a satisfaction that only God can give. He can give that inner peace that many search for, whether they know it or not.

Holy Joe

The Lord must become real in your heart. You must have information that becomes a revelation. I myself had to be informed about what the will of God was for me and then had to apply it to my life. Let me explain.

All my life I believed in Jesus and the Bible but I did not know that I needed Jesus in my heart. I didn't know Romans 10:9, which told me that if I confess the Lord Jesus with my mouth and believe in my heart that God raised Him from the dead, then I would be saved.

Over twenty years ago, while waiting for a truck to take me from Da Nang to a base camp, I sat with my pack, everything I owned in the world. When I looked down at the ground, I found this little pamphlet called "Holy Joe."

It was a picture track about this Holy Joe who joined the service. His sergeant was hard on him and tried to break him with very hard work. But the harder the sergeant got with him, the harder Joe worked. Joe tried to tell everyone about the

Bible and Jesus. Everyone made fun of him and called him names. Later they all went to war and the sergeant sent Joe on a very dangerous mission. Joe was killed and when the sarge found out, he repented and gave his life to the Lord. Then the sergeant was killed and the tract showed him on judgment day that he went to heaven. He had taken information and made it revelation.

Oh, I'll never forget reading that tract. It was the first time I ever read anything on how to get saved. I always thought I was okay. For some reason I thought that if I was nice and tried to help people, then I would go to heaven. I never read the Bible and never knew the truth about Jesus. But, there I was, in Vietnam, reading a tract someone had left there. Can you imagine it? Someone sent that tract to Vietnam over twenty years ago. I don't know who sent it or to whom it was sent, but God made sure it was there, just for me.

Because of that tract and someone's obedience in sending it, a seed was planted in my heart and I understood the plan of salvation. I thought about it for days. I knew deep in my heart, for the first time, that I was not right with God. I began to ask Jesus to help me, save me and protect me. Time and time again He did.

I remember being pinned down for hours with bullets flying right over our heads. One time we were pinned down in a rice paddy. That night, still soaking wet, we wondered just how close the bullets had come. When we took off our canteens that were strapped around our waists, they were full of bullet holes. We were only inches from being seriously wounded. It was there I made a covenant with God. I told Him I would serve Him in any way He wanted. I believe the Lord heard that prayer and started me on the journey of faith.

Here I am now, over twenty years later and I see how the Lord had His hand on me all this time. I challenge you to look back and examine the times the Lord put opportunities in your life and the times you knew God had His hand upon you. Somewhere you might have met a real "Holy Joe" who tried to tell you God's plan of salvation for your life. Think back, and realize it is God calling you to Him.

Like the story of the prodigal son in Luke 15, the father waited for his son to come home. The father, when he saw the son coming, ran to him and covered him with love. So too is our Heavenly Father waiting for you to come to Him. Make that move of faith and hear the Father say, "Welcome Home."